In Vitro

IN VITRO

ON LONGING AND TRANSFORMATION

ISABEL ZAPATA

Translated by Robin Myers

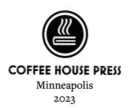

COFFEE HOUSE PRESS
Minneapolis
2023

First English-language edition published 2023
Copyright © 2021 by Isabel Zapata
Translation © 2023 by Robin Myers
Illustrations © Alejandro Magallanes
Cover artwork © Jimena Estíbaliz
Cover design by Zoe Norvell
Book design by Ann Sudmeier
Author photograph © Nuria Lagarde

First published by Almadía as *In Vitro*, © 2021

Coffee House Press books are available to the trade through our primary distributor, Consortium Book Sales & Distribution, cbsd.com or (800) 283-3572. For personal orders, catalogs, or other information, write to info@coffeehouse press.org.

Coffee House Press is a nonprofit literary publishing house. Support from private foundations, corporate giving programs, government programs, and generous individuals helps make the publication of our books possible. We gratefully acknowledge their support in detail in the back of this book.

LIBRARY OF CONGRESS CATALOGING-IN-PUBLICATION DATA

Names: Zapata, Isabel, 1984– author. | Myers, Robin, 1987– translator.
Title: In vitro / Isabel Zapata ; translated by Robin Myers.
Other titles: In vitro. English
Description: First English-language edition. | Minneapolis : Coffee House Press, 2023. |
Identifiers: LCCN 2022042755 (print) | LCCN 2022042756 (ebook) | ISBN 9781566896757 (paperback) | ISBN 9781566896764 (epub)
Subjects: LCSH: Zapata, Isabel, 1984-—Health. | Fertilization in vitro, Human—Mexico—Anecdotes. | Fertilization in vitro, Human—Psychological aspects—Anecdotes. | Pregnancy—Mexico—Anecdotes. | Pregnancy—Psychological aspects—Anecdotes. |Parental grief—Mexico—Anecdotes.
Classification: LCC RG135 .Z3713 2023 (print) | LCC RG135 (ebook) | DDC 618.1/780599—dc23/eng/20221122
LC record available at https://lccn.loc.gov/2022042755
LC ebook record available at https://lccn.loc.gov/2022042756

Katsushika Hokusai, "The Great Wave off Kanagawa" image courtesy of the Metropolitan Museum of Art, online database entry 45434.

María Auxiliadora Álvarez, excerpt from "Cuerpo (4)" from *Cuerpo/Ca(z)a*. Copyright © 1993 by María Auxiliadora Álvarez. Reprinted with the permission of the author. Translated by Robin Myers.

Natalie Shapero, excerpt from "Survive Me" from *Hard Child*. Copyright © 2017 by Natalie Shapero. Reprinted with the permission of The Permissions Company, LLC on behalf of Copper Canyon Press, coppercanyonpress.org.

PRINTED IN THE UNITED STATES OF AMERICA

30 29 28 27 26 25 24 23   1 2 3 4 5 6 7 8

For Aurelia, who trusted us with her name

Even before my body was an instrument for language it had been an instrument for memory.

Sarah Manguso

Writing also means not speaking. Keeping silent. Screaming without sound.

Marguerite Duras

Translator's Note

When I first read *In Vitro*, I felt it: a crack, a delicate fissure opened as if by a swift blow on rock, then the rushing in of something big and bright. I wasn't ready.

For months, I had felt—this was well into the first year of the COVID-19 pandemic—unable to feel much at all, at least not with any precision. And for months, even years before that, I'd been lurching in and out of my own desire to become a parent, and my fear, and the tangle of other feelings that sometimes exasperated and sometimes anguished and sometimes eluded me altogether. At the time of this writing, I haven't yet unraveled the snarl. And so, when Isabel Zapata's book arrived in my inbox and I began to read, it wasn't so much that I identified with the stories it tells as I felt instantly exposed to them, vulnerable to what they might stir up in me. I wept in a way I hadn't for a long time.

I'm allowing myself to share these thoughts as an accompaniment to *In Vitro* because they accompanied, in an unusual way, my process of translating it. Unusual for me, I mean: I generally experience translation as an act of intimacy but not catharsis, approaching even a text I love with an almost clinical sense of curiosity. Not quite detachment, but certainly distance. I'm aware of where the language ends and I begin. My job is to follow that language, let it show me how it works; I'm not usually swimming in it, soaked to the bone. With *In Vitro*, feeling as raw and porous as I did, I knew I would need to work harder and more slowly to find my footing. It was in her craft that I would find it, in the structural and tonal elements that shaped the voice I found so moving: a voice both yearning and contained, hard-edged but gestural, unsparing, rapt.

Zapata is a poet, too, and everything I admire most about her poetry is also present in her prose. A clean, smooth line that often swerves somewhere unexpected. A stride both methodical and spontaneous. A keen attention to nonhuman lives and presences. A graceful interlacing of other writers' work into her own. An unblinkingness. That's a lot of it: reading Zapata, I feel like I'm looking through the eyes of someone who isn't afraid to look steadily, and for a long time, at something uncomfortable enough that many others would rather glance away. This is an affective consequence of her writing, but it's rooted in style. Her pace, her register, her prosody.

Translating *In Vitro* was a continual exercise in paring down. Sometimes an image came to mind unbidden: someone whittling a block of wood into a fish. Let the record show that I don't know the first thing about fish-whittling, but the picture kept flashing back to me as I worked: the carving, the shavings, the improbable flick of a tail. How could I make my English both hard and supple? What could I get rid of to make a line feel crisper and more sure of itself, whether it was driving forth into certainty or veering out into the lack of it?

Ultimately, I read *In Vitro* as a book about uncertainty: an exploration, frank and streaked with wonder, of the places in a person's life where longing meets grief, where the world's harsh upheaval meets the tenderness of living here, where the joy of being someone's daughter or mother never eliminates—only accompanies—the loss, the strangeness, the eternal unresolvability of it all. Reading and translating this book has not answered my own questions. Somehow, though, it has strengthened them—or strengthened me as I hold them close, where they belong.

Robin Myers
Mexico City, June 2022

In Vitro

The Great Wave

I write these words without knowing whether anyone else will ever read them. The only person I've shared them with so far—a man—said they made him feel like an intruder. What kind of intruder am I speaking to? Shyly, I alternate certain fragments with other people's stories so I can say I'm writing a work of fiction. It's my house, but other women walk the halls.

The truth lives somewhere inside what I'm telling you here, but memory isn't what leads us to the truth. Not really.

It's hard to identify the most important parts of this story. I'm telling what happened to me, what happened to my body and to me, to my daughter's body and to my body and to me, but every time I remember it, I transform it. That's why I tell it in the present tense, but by taking steps backward, like someone leaving her beloved after they've said goodbye, unwilling to look away. Whenever I try to reduce my narrative to the basics, tiny details swell with meaning: on the day of the transfer, the doctor wore a pair of ruby-red-framed glasses that made her look like a fantastical bird. I cut myself more than once by breaking vials of progesterone. I still have the disposable robe I stole from the examining room. I want to say everything and know everything and hear everything. I want to shatter the vow of silence that isolates the painful parts of motherhood. I'm raising my voice so that the story can take on a life of its own and find its place in the company of other women.

I release it. I release myself.

In Vitro

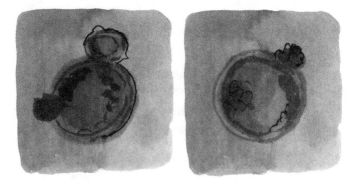

My first thought when the doctor shows me an image of the two embryos he's about to insert into my body is that the one on the left is the rebellious sibling, impatient to shake off its membrane. The proper name for the doctor in question is *embryologist*: a biologist specialized in morphogenesis, which means the development of embryos and nervous systems from gametogenesis to the birth of living beings. I smile at him, but his expression remains stern.

At this point, I decide to strip the embryos of all human features. They're recently unfrozen zygotes with just five days of development behind them: a cluster of cells. If I call them zygotes, it's easier to keep from thinking of the rebellious sibling, which looks eager to flee the place where it's spent eight weeks freezing to death. I correct myself again: they can't freeze to death if they've never been alive. So why is the rebellious sibling in such a rush to get out?

If we have twins, I'll bet the left embryo will take after Santiago, who can never sit still, and the right one after me, as I often wait around for longer than I'd like. That's what I'm thinking when the nurse asks me to drink another glass of water and change into my robe so we can start the procedure. The word *procedure* has nothing to do with my brimming bladder, the gun-shaped speculum, the progesterone injections that stamp an atlas of bruises across my ass, or my endometrium as it struggles to attain the ideal eight millimeters of thickness.

My psychoanalyst begins our session by saying that the desire to be a mother isn't the same as the desire to have a child. I turn the idea over and over, but I can't seem to wrap my head around it. So for the next forty-five minutes, I divide my childhood into compartments, as if life were a wardrobe and my memories were different garments to arrange by color. To figure out why I've gotten myself into this situation, I try to stir up experiences I've repressed for years. Maybe everything I say is true, maybe not, but that's not really the point: in psychoanalysis, events matter less than how we remember them.

In the process, I talk about things that don't make much sense and others that sound artificial, projected, like the script of a movie I wouldn't even watch on Netflix on a rainy Sunday night when I have nothing better to do. Psychoanalysis is a set, a stage, a radical unfolding. On the divan, my feet resting on a soft blanket I wish I could wrap around myself, I observe myself speaking, unable to recognize myself in my own words, blurting out sentences as if I were in a hurry. Everything about my speech feels foreign to me: I'm a river that doesn't know anything about the slope that governs it. When I hesitate, Fernando urges me to continue without trying too hard to organize my thoughts. The source of language—and psychoanalysis is, after all, the talking cure—isn't logic. It's imagination.

When I was younger, I thought motherhood began when you left the hospital with a baby swaddled in your arms. I figured there wouldn't be much to worry about until then, that pregnancy was mostly a question of buying miniature clothes and rubbing your belly with essential oils. Now I struggle to picture the scenes that once flashed before me of their own accord. A baby, which then seemed to me like an origin, now feels more like an end.

The beginning isn't the baby, it's the egg.

The nurse inserts a set of metal stirrups into the surgical bed and asks me to spread my legs and support them there. Then she drapes me with a blue cloth that covers my entire body, except for a hole that leaves my vulva exposed. Through an abdominal ultrasound, she evaluates the position of my uterus and the state of my endometrium, then conducts a deep cervical cleaning. A few minutes later, the doctor bustles in, announcing that one of the embryos wants out. *The rebellious sibling,* I think, but I don't say it.

The embryo transfer itself doesn't require sedation, but I feel absolutely narcotized: hope is a powerful drug. The operating room is dark except for the lamp shining directly between my legs. I don't see the embryologist approaching with a metal tray in his hands, like a scene from a horror movie, and I don't hear him, either: I need to pee so desperately that my ears hum. The cannula advances swiftly toward my uterus, but I don't realize that the embryos are inside until the nurse points to a tiny dot on my endometrium, projected on the screen behind me. Before she leaves, the doctor wishes me luck and gives me a hug that feels sincere.

Back in the cubicle, as I wait the mandatory half hour before I can go to the bathroom, Santiago tries to distract me. But every time he says *cannula* I think *urinal* and my bladder starts to throb. I pick up my cell phone and Google *ivf what happens if i pee.* The first article informs me that the transfer is conducted by means of a *quick, simple, and painless* procedure. Worse: it's *a special and exciting moment.* Fed up, I put down the device and yell that if someone doesn't come in soon I'm going to piss myself on the examining table. Then I think about the ten weeks of injections ahead of me, and will I get pregnant or won't I, and what would it be like to have twins, and what are we going to do with the other two frozen embryos if we don't end up using them. When I'm finally allowed to go to the bathroom, I relax: in a sudden fit of cheer, I think that the embryologist will be kind to them.

We already have hopes and beliefs about you, and we deposit them into your ghost before you exist, not even knowing if you will exist. It's cheating, I know: writing these things, using you as a recipient. The worst kind of deceit. An easy device, like when my mother died and I'd fall asleep fuming aloud, airing my grievances to her. That's what's left of my grief: the fear of forgetting her voice.

You don't yet have a voice, but sometimes I can hear it.

From the moment we begin to gestate in our mothers' wombs, women's bodies carry a finite number of eggs. If a woman gives birth to a girl, she also gives birth to the eggs that may make her a grandmother someday. The germinal cells in a few-weeks-old embryo already contain the genetic material of several future generations: the ability of one generation to create another. An embryo's primary mandate isn't to make a heart or a liver or four limbs with all their fingers and toes intact; it's just to *make more*.

I inhabit this hall of mirrors during the days of ovarian stimulation, wondering which of my reflections I should jab until the skin around my navel is stamped with tiny circles. The circles multiply with me: my womb is a lunar landscape glimpsed through purple glasses.

In vitro is an exercise in patience.

Among my family's myths about my mother is the tooth-paste myth, in which she realized she was pregnant the day after conceiving my two brothers and me. There were seven years between each of us. She knew because of the toothpaste: it tasted different. My mom was also a person who interpreted the transit of celestial bodies, hugged trees, handcrafted amulets using strange medieval charms, and spoke aloud to archangels, so I mocked her theories for years. Until the morning when I paused to study the minty taste in my mouth.

In 1932, Freud wrote to Einstein, *It may perhaps seem to you as though our theories are a kind of mythology and, in the present case, not even an agreeable one. But does not every science come in the end to a kind of mythology like this? Cannot the same be said to-day of your own Physics?*

As far as origins and endings are concerned, we have only myths, like the one I'm trying to create as I write. Anyone who wants meticulously recounted procedures and incontestable results will have to look elsewhere.

In the first essay of *Somos luces abismales* (We're lights in the abyss), Carolina Sanín says that if her dog could speak, she'd surely call her owner "I." Isn't that a little like having a child—a creature who takes months to understand that her mother isn't actually part of her? An organ that detaches from its body and starts wandering around, as if that were the most natural thing in the world?

I've never felt a love less ambivalent than the love I feel for my dog, but I have no idea what she feels. I know she wants to be with me all the time; that she likes soft tortillas, grass, sun, and walks; and that I give her all of those things. Isn't it a kind of parenthood when I explain to her that if it's raining and we're indoors, the rain can't hurt her? Aren't my dog and I—haven't we been for years now—a family? Her existence, her unshatterable company, is the closest thing I know to having a place in the world. To being someone's world. Or maybe love is always selfish in the end: I need her because she protects me from disintegration.

After the fertilization process, which takes place in the clinic, miles from my apartment, we're presented with a table: the history of each egg obtained by follicular aspiration. Of the fifteen follicles readied by ovarian stimulation, eight eggs were extracted and inseminated: four of them by "natural" means (the irony doesn't escape me) and four by intracytoplasmic sperm injection—ICSI—that places the sperm directly inside the egg with a micro-needle. Seven were fertilized: three of those were discarded in the subsequent hours and four were frozen, ready for transfer. Fate: viable.

Egg number	Type of fertilization	Embryonic development					
		Day 2	Day 3	Cellular symmetry	Fate	Day 5	Fate
1	ICSI	4c	8c	Yes	Sequential	BE (b/b)	Freeze
2	ICSI	4c	8c	No	Sequential	BC (b/bc)	Freeze
3	ICSI	4c	7c	No	Sequential	BQ	Not viable
4	ICSI	5c	7c	No	Sequential	BQ	Not viable
5	IVF	4c	10c	No	Sequential	BE (b/b)	Freeze
6	IVF	4c	8c	No	Sequential	BE (b/b)	Freeze
7	IVF	4c	8c	No	Sequential	BQ	Not viable

Several days after the transfer, I start taking progesterone injections to prepare my body. You can buy the substance, unsettlingly dubbed "yellow body strong," at any pharmacy; at mine, a woman administers the injection in the back office. She seems to dislike me, maybe because I'm tense and irritable on arrival and don't breathe deeply or relax or sit still when she asks me to.

To prepare my body, I wrote, but what I really mean is *to trick it.* The progesterone makes my body believe it's pregnant from day one—when the eggs are inseminated in a lab—to day five, when the transfer occurs. That's what lots of gynecological treatments are about, from contraceptives to assisted reproduction: they force the body to do what it wouldn't naturally be doing. They intervene.

The body is such a ruthless enemy that it's best to have it on our side.

On the afternoon before the transfer, we call the clinic to decide which embryos will be unfrozen at eleven the next morning. According to the table we'd received, our options are numbers one, two, five, and six; three are classified as B (normal quality) and one as C (poor quality). The embryologist recommends we try one and five (number one is the rebellious sibling). When I ask him if there's any risk involved in transferring non-excellent embryos, he says no: some are better than others, but none of them are defective. We choose the two he recommends and I hang up, hands trembling.

I scour the internet for the worst possible experiences, hunting for persuasive arguments against my plans. I'm my own devil's advocate. I spend hours on forums where women all over the world warn one another about the possible risks of the medications sitting on my bureau, describe their own repeatedly thwarted attempts, and mull over the next steps: trying again with donor eggs, adopting, moving on for their own peace of mind and accepting a childless future. Some even mention the possibility of a surrogate and lay out the conditions that every geographical region establishes for the exchange.

I observe from a distance, but I don't participate. Since the forums don't alert the other women to my presence, I'm like a gorilla wearing a hat and smoking a pipe as she studies the other gorillas through a glass cage at a zoo. I hope the other members of my species will recognize me as part of the group.

When the utilities receipt comes in the mail, I read *water birth* instead of *water bill*.

In vitro is an exercise in hallucination.

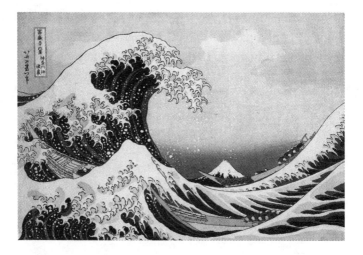

One of the first gifts I ever gave Santiago was a magnet of Hokusai's *The Great Wave off Kanagawa*. I bought it in a museum and presented it to him after a trip, along with a postcard in which I told him I loved him so much it was like drowning in that wild crest and other things too sappy to repeat. Soon after, an earthquake brought the city to its knees and our love, flighty and erratic and delirious as it was, became our only certainty in the face of disaster. It was crazy, getting married; at the same time, it felt like the only sensible step we could take. That was the tone of another decision we made two years later: to undergo the first embryo transfer one Friday afternoon when the Mexico City air was even more staggeringly polluted than usual. Its own version of the end of the world.

Sometimes I fantasize about having the embryologist over for dinner so Santiago can impress him with his couscous, like the first time we ate together at his apartment: the night of couscous with olives, of dream-catcher under-wear, of our transformation into Italian actors smoking in Tuscany.

That first night, we cooked with bloodied hands.

We read the future in the moisture stains on the ceiling.

The next day, a nest with six blue eggs appeared in the bromeliad out back.

My mother and aunt and I met Maricela in Havana in 1998. She was sitting in Cathedral Square with her hair in a red bandanna, skinny legs dangling from her flowered dress like a pair of black threads. It was impossible to guess her age, although she soon told us that she was over ninety. I'd just turned fourteen, and it was painfully obvious: my body was spindly, lumpy, disproportionate. When my mom told her I hadn't gotten my period yet—we barely knew her, but she often blurted out this kind of information unprovoked—Maricela looked at me intently, her brow furrowed, and urged me to never wash my underwear at the laundromat or hang it up to dry where strangers could see it. Her tone of voice suggested that this was a matter of life and death.

From Havana, we were headed for Trinidad, and Maricela gave us a parting gift: some colorful beaded necklaces that my mother immediately put on. For the rest of our trip, over patacones and mojitos, people stared at her hard. Later I learned that they were Santería necklaces; by wearing them, my mother was transmitting a message she was oblivious to and I haven't dared investigate.

Years later, when neither she nor my mother nor the Havana of 1998 existed anymore, I lived in a city where a personal washing machine was a luxury I couldn't afford. And so, for six long years, I washed my underwear exclusively in coin-operated laundries shared with dozens, perhaps hundreds, of strangers.

When I still hadn't started menstruating by my fifteenth birthday, my mother took me to see Dr. V., who diagnosed me with polycystic ovary syndrome and prescribed contraceptives to counteract the symptoms. For the eighteen years he was my gynecologist, this white-haired, ascot-wearing man never bothered to tell me that cysts are simply follicles—would-be eggs, would-be children—and not the little clods of grime I imagined inside me. He also failed to mention that the pills I'd swallow every night for the next eighteen years were designed to keep my body from ovulating, or that, when I wanted to get pregnant, I'd have to give my reproductive system the opposite command: a swerve so violent I'd struggle to recognize myself in the mirror.

I don't tell anyone about our plans because I hate getting asked how it's going. It embarrasses me to describe the procedures I'm inflicting on my body. Some things remain unsaid. Or else you say them only in a low voice, only to your closest friends, always in euphemisms, as if our hands were sullied by paying to reproduce. *We're in treatment.* How's it going? The answer is always the same, *not well,* and the repetition feels like rewatching a movie that bored you the first time.

At the end of one of our last appointments, Dr. V. says my nerves are the problem, that I need "to give my crazy head a rest." All I have to do is relax, he insists, looking steadily at Santiago. In one fell swoop, he disqualifies my experience and erases me both from the examining room and from my own exhausted body.

By this point, we've had regular appointments with him for almost a year. His diagnosis was clear from day one: we're struggling to conceive because of my hormonal disorder. At first, he suggested we try timed intercourse, a treatment that involves conducting controlled ovarian stimulation and then, once one or two follicles measure at least eighteen millimeters in diameter, administering a dose of gonadotropin-releasing hormone that causes ovulation between thirty-four and thirty-eight hours later: which is exactly when you're supposed to have sex. But the most fertile moment of an induced cycle is also the most painful one, which makes sex its polar opposite. If the point of fucking is to dissolve the boundaries imposed by the flesh and attain something like unity, timed intercourse is a reminder of what keeps us apart.

We visited Dr. V.'s examining room every week for months. The follicles grew, the eggs were released, and intercourse was carried out according to plan, but the blood flowed punctual and abundant as never before. When he saw that his treatment wasn't working, the doctor increased the hormone dose, and before he even considered having Santiago undergo a semen analysis, he suggested piercing my ovaries with an electric scalpel. Dr. V. assumed Santiago was fine, since he was young and healthy. But wasn't I young and healthy, too?

Teetering on the edge of burnout, I often wanted to tell the doctor to seek the problem elsewhere, but I never said a word. It's a silence that still haunts me today. I was paralyzed by the thought of contradicting him.

When I left that office forever, I exercised my right to live a bearable life and pursue the conditions for our family to continue, to move on.

I must inform you that it's all a wound these days, writes Gonzalo Rojas, which is a little like what these pages feel like for me: the wound as a perversion, an unnatural inclination, an alteration of reality.

The Etruscans butchered animals to read the future in their entrails.

I seek my fortune in a petri dish.

I spend my birthday in bed with ovarian hyperstimulation syndrome: an overdose of the hormones prescribed by Dr. V. My ovaries feel swollen and my belly looks like I've had a balloon inflated inside me. Short of breath, unable to move half an inch without feeling like my uterus is rupturing, I cancel the cake and lie motionless for hours. When I get up to pee, I collapse onto the floor. Santiago grabs his phone and calls the doctor, who sounds worried for the first time since I've known him. He tells me not to move around much, prescribes industrial quantities of painkillers, and asks for hourly updates. If I'm not better soon, he warns, I'll need an emergency operation. I spend the next two weeks vomiting out of sheer repulsion, my womb empty of embryos.

In Vitro

you've never given birth

you've never known
machete blades

you haven't felt
the river snakes

you've never danced
in a pool of beloved blood

doctor

don't reach your hand too far inside
that's where I keep the blades
that's where I've got a sleeping girl
and sir, you've never spent
a night inside the snake
you've never known the river

I want to give birth so I can live inside this poem by María Auxiliadora Álvarez. So I can dance in a pool of beloved blood. So I can meet the river. So I can be sure I'm more like her than the doctor who speaks of flesh but has never sharpened machetes with his own hands.

I put the image of the embryos on the refrigerator when I get home. I feel like a character in a scene from a Hollywood romantic comedy: predictable, cliché, determined to make my life into one of those scenes where a little boy runs into the kitchen with a sheet of paper in his hand—almost always a drawing of a house and a sun and a happy stick-figure family—and throws his arms around the legs of his mother, who smiles and immediately hangs up the drawing for everyone to see.

So we won't forget, I tell myself. As if we could.

Some nights, as I wash dishes or take out ingredients for dinner, I stop and stare at the embryos for a long time. When I see my full name sitting on a corner of the paper beside the clinic logo, the word *patient* takes on a new meaning.

I decide to leave Dr. V. a year after I started the treatment that poisoned me. Fed up with allopathic medicine, I see an iridologist who searches my eyes for lines, blotches, and discolorations, anything that might suggest a pathological imbalance, and mixes magic potions to reverse them. His techniques may sound dubious, but at this point I find them far more reasonable than continually injecting myself with chemicals I can't even pronounce. In addition to daily herbs, he gives me some special tea in a brown paper bag and prescribes a purge with simple steps to follow over the weekend.

I drink the tea early on Saturday morning. The cramps don't start for hours. When they do, they take me by storm. I shit and vomit objects of totally inexplicable origin: strips of charred cloth, layers of old mucus, shreds of scab and flesh. As if someone had crammed my intestines with gauze at birth and forgotten to take it out.

That night I dream of snakes shedding their skin.

I start to bleed on Sunday night.

The first thing Dr. B. asks us is why Santiago hasn't had any tests done—part of the clinical analyses that follow any diagnosis of infertility in a heterosexual couple. When we tell her that our previous doctor didn't think it was necessary, she lowers her eyes and prescribes those tests as a first step in any subsequent treatment. She jots something brief in my file. I'd love to know what it says.

A few days later, we show up at an immaculately white-walled laboratory that looks like the inside of an abandoned spaceship. A nurse calls Santiago's name and gives him a series of instructions I'm not close enough to overhear. It's not my place to tell what happens next.

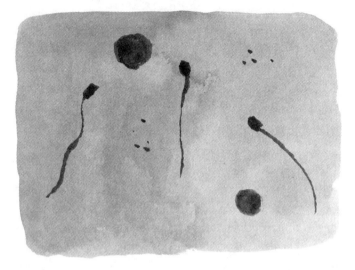

The night we get the results of the spermatobioscopy, we go to a party—not because there's any good news to celebrate, but because it's a friend's birthday and one of our ironclad pacts is that we won't let the treatment interfere with normal life. And normal life means going to our friends' birthday parties. On beer number five, Santiago takes the test results out of his backpack and marches around the apartment, euphoric, showing off the image of his semen. "I'm as sterile as a broomstick! Today the myth of Santiago the Stud has crumbled!" he crows, relishing his own comic genius. I go for a gin and tonic and return to the couch, where I entertain myself by watching strangers' faces react to the unexpected sight of my husband's scant, misshapen spermatozoa.

Sometimes I think that life is a gift with a catch. It's a mediocre gift, or at least a selfish one, because I give it to myself through you.

Is it too late to change my mind?

A few months after my mother's death, when I was twenty years old, her friend Javier dreamed I was pregnant with a baby girl in which my mother would supposedly be reincarnated. The image consoled me: my mother was coming back, it was just a matter of time. Soon I'd be the one responsible for giving birth to her, nursing her, changing her diapers, showing her how sunlight hits certain objects, shining until it hurts them.

After the transfer, we let two weeks pass, known as the "beta wait," to see if either of the embryos has been implanted successfully. I try not to think about it: I fill my hours with work and coffee dates, my dog walks grow longer, my unstructured time compresses. I set myself ridiculous tasks, like removing all the clothes from my closet, folding them, and putting them back. Checking the expiration dates of all the medications in the bathroom cabinet. Organizing my Word documents in order of importance.

For those two weeks, I sit myself down before the blank screen because I can't find anywhere else to be. My body isn't brief, it's abbreviated.

The first image that appeared when I Googled *Leticia city Colombia* was a statue of some pink dolphins undulating among the palm trees. Undulating, too, is the brand-new life of Leticia, my niece. Two days after her birth, my brother texted me *Leticia has knees!!!* and my phone has been full of baby photos ever since. Leticia curled up on the scale in the hospital with a little tag around her foot, or playing with a rattle from Oaxaca, her arm extended like Buzz Lightyear: to infinity and beyond!

I especially remember a picture taken when she was just four or five months old, which my brother juxtaposed with one of me at the same age. We were identical. Flooded with hormones, I rankled at the resemblance. I cried for several days until the night I collapsed in a panic on the living room couch. Soon after, discussing the meltdown with my psychoanalyst, I tell him that I have a newborn niece who looks a lot like me.

"I could be that baby," I say in a tragic voice.

"What would you say is the biggest difference between the two of you?"

I respond without hesitation: "I'm an orphan and she isn't."

If Leticia is the little girl in the dream, the one my mother's friend had, then who will come back to life in my daughter's body?

On the fifth day after the transfer, I have lunch with a friend I rarely see. He takes a seat across from me and immediately recognizes a tattoo I'd gotten a couple years before: "Is that the pool at your dad's house?" he asks, even though it's an abstract drawing and the sketch is so poorly executed that the line blurs on my left forearm. Isn't this the closest thing to sharing a language with someone else?

For years, I was tortured by the thought that my children would never know my mother: a hurt that bound non-existent people together. I imagined them playing with her long witchy necklaces, sliding a loaf of banana bread into the oven, listening to her go on about astronomical conjunctions in a library that's been closed for fifteen years and yet lives on in me. But the pain softened over time, and now I can't even picture my mother as a grandmother. She still has the shoulder-length golden hair she had when I was a little girl. She wears plaid shirts and jackets with corduroy elbow patches (to pass for a professor, she says). She carries the extra pounds that the cancer plucked from her frame. There are no medications in sight, just books and half-drunk coffee cups and multicolored beads. She's a woman with an entire pancreas, an unscathed stomach, an open future: haughty, brilliant, myopic, beautiful, glimmering. My mother is always young in my dreams.

We're in Acapulco, about to take a boat to Isla de la Roqueta. We came because a friend told us it was gorgeous there, but we instantly realize that her recommendation was a little over the top. It takes us half an hour to board the boat because a teenager insists on selling us a whole tour, which includes a visit to the virgin of the sea and a fish show that basically consists of peering into the boat's glass bottom to watch sea creatures as they swim. And off we go, glimpsing the flutters of fish fins through murky glass. Everything reminds me of embryos.

I've been steering clear of "women's issues" for ages without really knowing what they are and almost certainly failing to avoid them altogether. Deep down, the phrase makes me squirm because women's issues don't exist: there are issues and there are people and everyone writes about whatever they want. Except motherhood, which, on second thought, may well be a women's issue, but I'm not yet allowed to write about it. At the end of the day, this is actually a ghost story.

We all loved Santa, a German shepherd puppy so obedient that she was born already trained, as my mother would say. Guillermina, our live-in housekeeper, loved her the most. She'd fix delicacies for Santa out of chicken guts, rice, and tortilla scraps; she'd walk her every morning; in the evenings, she'd sit at the kitchen table and brush her with a patience we didn't have.

One morning, Santa suddenly fell sick and died that same night. It happened as things always happened in my childhood, which was like a stage with characters who entered and exited without warning or explanation: one day the dog just wasn't there anymore. Guillermina seemed distracted all weekend, her gaze remote. On Monday, when I came downstairs for breakfast, her bags were packed and waiting by the door. That night, my mother said she'd been rummaging around in the laundry room and discovered some rodenticide. Then she found a little altar in Guillermina's room, arranged with flowers and lit candles and photos of both Antonio—her son—and Santa.

It took me almost thirty years to understand, but now I believe that her motives weren't entirely cruel. Antonio, who had died in an accident at the age of fourteen, never knew what it was like to love a dog, and his mother feared that no one would help him across the lands of the dead. Our puppy had been poisoned.

Here, Guillermina. Take Santa. I'm giving her to you. (A baby wouldn't have the strength to help me across the river.)

Speaking of ghosts, some women catch the scent of their dead mothers as they nurse their children.

During the first seven days after fertilization, the embryo cells multiply in the outer membrane of the oocyte, a tiny jumble of powder and proteins, until they grow so large that they break right through and embed themselves in the inner layer of the uterus. Frozen ones spend their early days in straw pipettes, stored in tanks of liquid nitrogen at -321°F, a temperature that halts all biological activity and keeps their physiology intact. To prevent potentially harmful ice crystals from forming, antifreezing substances called cryoprotectants are applied.

It's best not to use the word *life* when thinking about this process. Saying that the embryos *live* in the ice, or that they spend their first *days of life* on a pipette, would radically transform the world I've built. Words aren't the map we use to travel the territory; they are the territory.

Another myth: one evening, when I was six years old, my mother asked me why I was crying disconsolately in the closet. I told her I was worried about what my eight future children would have to endure. I don't remember the incident in detail, but I do recognize that girl in the woman I've become: apprehensive, teeming with hang-ups and little obsessions. I recognize her habit of anticipatory distress.

My dog has almost died twice, as far as I know. The first time was shortly after she came to live with me. She wouldn't eat or drink, so I took her to the animal hospital, where a veterinarian told me she had distemper and there was nothing to be done. Since the treatment was expensive and recovery improbable, he recommended I have her euthanized. I refused.

For the two weeks she spent at the vet's, I was allowed to go in and see her briefly in the mornings and evenings, and I went every day, trying to establish contact with a creature I'd only just met. Many of the complex mechanisms of communication that now govern our shared life were forged during those visits, where I devoted myself to telling her why she had to stay in the hospital and to repeating her name aloud, so that the memory of the sound would protect her when she was alone. Before long, she came to understand that my visits would be constant and she began to expect them: after several days, one of the doctors told me she'd stand up and wag her tail a few minutes before my arrival. It was a simple matter of logic and punctuality.

Four days before the blood tests, a white noise of phone calls and deadlines drowns out the sound—so improbable that it hurts—of a curly-haired girl darting around the yard. If I reach out my hand, I can almost touch her, so I turn into a stone instead of a river: rigid, heavy, unwilling to change my course.

Isn't motherhood a way to disappear? Doesn't it force us to step aside?

I want to have a child so I can be made invisible.

A stone, says Eliot Weinberger, is hard and endures.
Which means it's in flux.

Sometimes we fantasize about how we'd spend the money it would have cost us to have a child if we don't manage to have one. Santiago insists parenthood is just one possible life among many others, and I play along when he launches into excitable monologues about the countries we'd visit, our house in paradise (ideally in Santa María Ahuacatitlán, Cuernavaca), the ten dogs we'd take hiking in Los Dinamos, a nature reserve near the city. Where I see disaster in the making, a limping life, he sees flights to Thailand, fruit trees, flapping puppy tongues.

My dog's second brush with death was due to giardia, an intestinal parasite. She was hospitalized for fewer days than the last time, but the conditions were worse: since she was contagious, no one could enter the room with her except to administer medication and check her vital signs. I didn't leave my apartment for several days, pacing from my room to the living room to the kitchen and back, helpless. Maybe, when I cried in the closet at age six, I was weeping for what my dogs would suffer in the future.

Five days after the embryo transfer, the only difference I sense in my body is a steep decline in my motor skills: I bruise my knees on the furniture, knock over glasses of water, collide with closed doors. It's as if I wanted to see things shatter, but I can't find the symptom on any website.

My mother's real surname doesn't exist. Or it's missing. The story changes depending on the relative who tells it, so I choose the version I like best: in which a Sephardic great-great-grandfather, one Gershom Zaragozí de la Horta by name, fled persecution in Spain, sailed to Mexico, and met Señorita Altagracia, whom he soon married. In which my great-grandfather Isaac was born in Atoyac, Jalisco, his surname already transmuted into Morales, which is the name he gave to his son Vicente, my grandfather, who passed it on to his daughter, Josefina, my mother, who spent years trying to reconstruct her Jewish family name. She didn't succeed, but she always kept a menorah on the table in the foyer.

In the documentary *Heart of a Dog*, Laurie Anderson describes a dream of giving birth to her dog Lolabelle. "It's almost a perfect moment," she says, "except that the joy is mixed with quite a lot of guilt."

The night before the blood work, I hit play on the mental movie that will run if I turn out to be pregnant. First, three months of silence in case of miscarriage. Will I want to hide the news from the four or five friends who have accompanied us through the process? Will I be able to? Then the series of tests to detect "anomalies": the clinical urine tests, the amniocentesis, the O'Sullivan test, the lung-maturity test, the fetal-DNA-in-maternal-blood test, the triple screen, the Doppler echocardiogram. Then the risks of birth, the postpartum period, the early years. To halt the onslaught of potential catastrophes, I remind myself of the success rate: less than 30 percent.

To the Greek poet Stesichorus, renowned for his epithets,
I wouldn't be the mother of babies, but the possessor of
embryos.

The acupuncturist pricks my body with tiny holes, then produces a syringe of procaine, an anesthetic. Would I mind if she injected it into the center of my thorax? she asks. Of course I mind, but I let her. I have a bruise the size of a ten-peso coin below my neck for the rest of the week. It shows, but no one asks me anything.

I take a walk with a friend to distract myself. When I tell him I'm nervous about the pregnancy test, he tries to reassure me. "If it doesn't work," he suggests, "just imagine that the kid would have looked like your least-favorite relative." What he doesn't say is that, if I do get pregnant, the possibility that the baby might resemble my least-favorite relative will become yet another thing to worry about.

Motherhood is a knife without a handle, says Nuria Labari in *La mejor madre del mundo* (The world's best mother). *You can't grab it without impaling yourself.*

The night before the pregnancy test, I dream I'm sitting on a toilet in my grandparents' house, which is nothing like their house in real life, and I'm in labor. I watch myself writhing, sweating, racked with pain. I spend hours like this. But the place keeps changing, like a theater set where the action continues while black-clothed stagehands replace the furniture as if no one can see them. When I finish and lean forward to see what I've expelled, I find myself confronted with two scraps of raw meat I identify as the embryos. Before I can thrust my hand into the bowl to save them, some god or spirit or force of nature flushes the toilet and I see them spiral away into the dark tube.

When Santiago and I argue for hours without getting any-where, I wonder whether a child might offer an alternate language, a sort of biological tether between two islands with radically different climates. Child as bridge. Then it occurs to me that the entire history of feminism—universal history, personal history, all of it—could be read as a warn-ing against this kind of thought.

Sleeping is something we learn in endless rehearsals, and the trance between wakefulness and slumber is so traumatic that some of us spend our childhoods trying to avoid it. In the end, the lesson is as simple as "fake it till you make it": close your eyes as if you were asleep, go to the office as if you liked your job, set the alarm as if you enjoyed going out for a run at seven a.m., talk to your womb until a child starts growing there.

One warm evening in June, the level of human chorionic gonadotropin in my blood (386) reveals five weeks of pregnancy.

Embryo

At my first appointment after the positive result, the doctor looks relieved to find just one gestational sac in the ultrasound (there's no way to tell if it's the rebellious sibling). By the five-week point, gastrulation has begun: the movement and migration of the simplest embryonic cells into the three primordial layers that will go on to produce the baby's tissues: the ectoderm or outer layer (nervous system, skin, and mouth), the mesoderm or middle layer (muscles, skeleton, circulatory system, reproductive system, and excretory system), and the endoderm or inner layer (lungs and organs of the digestive apparatus). The embryo's body curves slightly to one side and the blueprint of the heart now has three defined cavities, like the heart of a reptile.

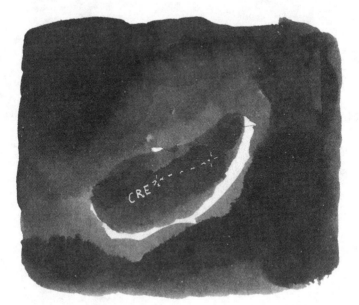

Before we leave, the nurse prints an image that shows a barely distinguishable yolk sac with the embryo inside, and she gives it to us: it's the first photograph we'll ever have of our baby, she says. But no: we already have the image of the two embryos we were given on the day of the transfer, five weeks before. When my daughter began to live outside me.

The first thing I do when we get home is replace the image of the embryos on the refrigerator with the photo of the yolk sac. Then I visit a website that calculates the probability of miscarrying based on the day of gestation, the mother's age, and the prior number of pregnancies that have resulted in a living baby. I have no idea how they come up with these figures, but the risk decreases over time: at exactly five weeks, at my age, weight, and height, the probability of losing the baby is 21.7 percent. At five weeks and three days, 19 percent. And two days later, it drops to 15 percent.

The page has another function that presents the probability not of losing the baby, but of carrying the pregnancy to term: the chance to see the glass half-full. The first day of the sixth week, that number clocks in at 85 percent. Beneath that figure appears the following sentence: "Since you got pregnant, your probability of miscarriage has dropped from approximately 39.9 percent to approximately 15 percent."

The miracle of finding no blood when I wipe myself after I pee is so astonishing that it demands measurement. And so I spend a lot of time changing the parameters—I imagine I'm twenty-five or forty, that I've already had two children or lost a baby at age twenty—to see how the probability of miscarrying is altered. I think about the women I could have been, but not with compassion. Deep down, there's something sinister about it: I'm listening for a voice to remind me that it could always be worse.

Money is no obstacle, I read in an ad for a fertility clinic. But it is. So much so that they give you your money back if you don't get pregnant within eighteen months. Age is also an obstacle. Otherwise there wouldn't be an entire section on the egg-freezing program *so you can pluck your star from the sky whenever you're ready.* The language is always roughly the same: dream, miracle, star from the sky. Yet the price tag, perhaps the most essential factor when it's time to make the call, is rarely revealed. According to a study of 372 clinics in the US, only 27 percent include a list of costs on their website.

That's not the only thing kept hidden. When transnational companies approach their top young female employees and offer financial plans so they can freeze their eggs and delay parenthood, they don't tell the women exactly what kinds of assisted reproductive treatments they'll have to undergo when they decide to become mothers, and they don't explain that the probability of such treatments actually resulting in a live baby plummet after age thirty-five. Despite the pastel-hued posters pinned up in fertility clinics and the technologies advancing in leaps and bounds, some people have negative test after negative test after negative test.

Elina Brotherus kept a log of the years she spent trying to get pregnant with the help of fertility treatments, from 2009 to 2013, through her photography project *Annonciation*. Various images in the series show her awaiting results more or less optimistically, surrounded by fresh flowers or calendars with the days crossed off. Others, though, depict the loss of what she never had: blood in the toilet bowl, her belly printed with bruises, wild visions of her impossible daughter, boxes of medications heaped up like a city and its outskirts (menotropin, Gonal-F, prednisone).

Hers is a story of false annunciations: the angel stands her up. In every failure, Brotherus says, the feeling is tantamount to grief, and the loss is vivid: "Not only does one lose a child, one also loses a whole future life as a family."

In *The Argonauts*, Maggie Nelson describes being a step-mother as an identity in tension. It wasn't until she had to confront the task of raising someone else's child, she says, that she was able to reflect on her stepfather's role in her own childhood. The thing is, it doesn't matter how wonderful, responsible, or loving you are: you'll always be susceptible to scorn. As someone who grew up with stepmothers and stepfathers all over the place, I accepted these stereotypes as true and didn't question them until many years later, when my family relationships had been warped by mountain ranges of resentment I couldn't even begin to traverse.

Esther Vivas, the author of *Mamá desobediente* (Disobedient mom), uses a term that could be translated as "kindred mother" to replace "stepmother," suggesting "reconstituted family" for families with children from previous marriages who suddenly become stepsiblings, stepchildren. Like my family, which became a sort of patchwork quilt: more than a reconstituted family, a family in a continual state of reconstitution. In the view of Sarah Hrdy, both mothers who give birth and mothers who adopt should be considered "biological mothers." Both, she writes, undergo similar neuroendocrinological transformations, even without the direct experience of labor or breastfeeding. A biological mother is the mother who nurtures, who nourishes, who provides the environment in which a child develops physically and biologically.

Words are alive, and, contrary to popular belief, they don't merely reflect the way we think; they're also the engine of ideas and actions. The entire world is contained inside them. Using one word instead of another entails a decision that transforms us. Doing away with certain prejudices about motherhood(s) necessarily calls for linguistic changes, too.

The clinic exists out of time. Here, reproductive technologies take colossal leaps forward in the controversial territories of embryo vitrification, endometrial scratching, gestational surrogacy, male pregnancy, and predetermining the sex of the fetus. I doubt I'll live long enough to see it, but as I wait for the nurse to call my name, I imagine an alternate reality in which it's possible to have a baby tailor-made: like ordering a drink in a coffee shop.

In the waiting room, I fight the urge to ask the other women how they got here, where they are in the process, how many eggs they've been able to fertilize, how they've handled the medications. The first rule of in vitro fertilization is to never talk about in vitro fertilization. If, in the veritable avalanche of books, blogs, and movies, it's difficult to find the voices of women who decided not to become mothers, finding the voices of those who wanted to but couldn't is practically impossible.

In November 2015, at the age of twenty, the Mexican artist Paola Livas finalized her donation of eleven eggs in exchange for monetary compensation amounting to fifteen thousand Mexican pesos, which she spent on school projects. In October, soon before the follicular aspiration that would conclude the process, she had second thoughts and tried to put an end to it. Ultimately, she wasn't allowed: in the nurse's words, she was already paired off. On the other side of the mirror, a woman was waiting for her eggs.

From that point onward, the possible life of her possible "non-child," as Livas calls it, began to haunt her. She bought onesies in markets and embroidered them with messages to her newborn ghost. She started a journal to document the effects of the hormones on her mood. (She still returns to it: it's a work in progress that bears some resemblance to a flesh-and-blood child.) Eventually, she traveled to a nearby town to collect a cradle she still has in her possession. The onesies, the journal, and the empty cradle have been put on exhibition several times as part of a piece she calls *Ficciones de la no-maternidad* (Fictions of non-motherhood).

Assuming that the pairing-off worked and one of her eggs enabled a conception in the same year those eggs were extracted from her, Paola's non-child is now five years old: her own age in the photograph she was asked to submit, along with a recent photo, when she began the donation paperwork. She's smiling in the portrait, dressed in bright-pink *Mulan* pajamas and a pair of bunny slippers. Sometimes, when she goes out for a walk, she studies little girls on the playground in search of that same beaming face.

When I tell a friend I'm afraid of showing up for my appointment and learning that the embryo doesn't have a heartbeat, she suggests I place a large glass against my belly and ask Santiago to listen through it.

I start to cry as soon as I hear the heart beating inside me and don't stop until we leave the clinic. One hundred thirty-eight beats per minute. It occurs to me that the embryo is on the verge of needing another name, ideally one that would describe its heartbeat, because that's practically all it is: a beating heart.

In the taxi back home, Santiago breaks the silence: "What's crazy is the rhythms are different. There are two hearts beating inside you, but each one has its own rhythm, like certain African drums." There's a kind of fascination in his voice. And a strong dash of envy.

In *Las nubes* (The clouds), Juan José Saer says a desert is identical to itself for leagues and leagues, in each and every one of its parts: only light interrupts the sensation of traveling continually along the very same stretch of space.

The light transforming the flatlands of my thirty-sixth year isn't the same light as always, repeated. It shines differently. It breaks with what used to be movement. It advances as if spilling over.

Yesterday a homeless man came up to me in the Colonia Roma and said you were a girl. It's not the first time I've been approached by a stranger on the street and pre-scribed my fortune. Maybe four years ago, a dark-skinned woman in a long skirt stopped me on Avenida Xola. "Do you remember me?" she asked, not waiting for an answer before she launched into a monologue about houses with fountains in the courtyards and birds dropping dead from the trees. She vanished into the crowd without asking for change or trying to sell me anything.

The man from yesterday said less. Although my belly is still flat, he guessed your presence with a single glance. A dot of light, as if he'd snapped an aura photo with his eyes alone. It's a girl, he said. In silence, he added: multiply. Multiply us.

The first baby ever conceived by in vitro fertilization was also a girl: Louise Joy Brown, born in Oldham, England, on July 25, 1978. Today, it's been calculated, somewhere between eight and ten million people have been born as a result of this procedure.

A dream: in the second ultrasound, the embryo is gone. The doctor picks up her prescription pad and writes: *escaped embryo, reexamine in three weeks.* Then she opens her desk drawer, takes out a can of red paint, dips a hand into it, and uses her fingers to sketch indecipherable signs across my belly. Before she leaves the office, she advises me to introduce rhinoceros meat into my diet—excellent for pregnant women.

Writing doesn't always lead to illumination. Sometimes it simply means you watch something turn into something else and confirm that everything is connected by invisible threads. While some of the experiences I'm narrating here have remained in the past, this story is revealing itself in real time, even for me. It's a letter written in lemon juice: to discover the secret message, you have to hold a lit match to it. Show it the existence of fire.

I lost my mother several months before her death and gained my daughter long before the day of her birth. We like to say that things happen in due time, and happen for a reason, but we're never actually prepared for anything.

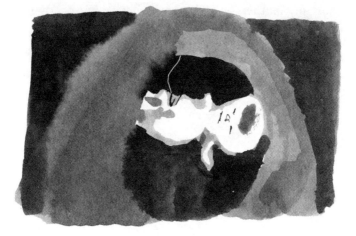

At twelve weeks, you're a set of circles arranged in order.

A water bear focused on its own repetition.

A voice aflame in darkness:
     black stone on a white stone,
     but the other way around.

What's the word that names you?
     blank page
     blank child

When I try to say your name, you turn into something else.
Like trying to catch a mosquito in your hand—without hurt-
ing it—in a dark room.

Medusa

I'm writing an exercise of future memory. I thread together the days, lived and unlived, to tell the story I want my jellyfish to remember once it's able to. Along the way, I also decide what I hope we'll both forget. I erase the feeling left by the sugar solution in my throat.

If a net is a swath of holes designed to catch just a fraction of the boundless ocean it plunges into, here, too, the blank space exceeds what is said. That's why these pages resist becoming a diary. They're more like a serial novel, an invention, a delicate clearing of the throat.

The first time I dream of you, you're already walking. Your hair is black and curly. You dance with your hands pressed into fists, swinging your hips back and forth. You're a girl, and from then on I refer to you in the feminine, despite the fact that everyone, except for the homeless man in the Colonia Roma and me, is convinced you're a boy.

Five minutes after the nine-week ultrasound, the doctor tells us about the screening test for Down syndrome and other chromosomal abnormalities. It involves another ultrasound and a blood test. The first turns out fine. A few days later, though, the doctor calls about the blood results: they show that our baby has a high risk of possessing an extra copy of the twenty-first chromosome. We'll need to do a more exacting diagnostic test.

I'm at a friend's house when I get the call. In someone else's bathroom, then, I press my hands to the mirror and try to keep from crying out. *Expecting* is the term that best describes pregnancy: joy mixed with the constant anticipation of ghost movies, when the main character tiptoes down a dark corridor, expecting a specter to strike. Fear becomes the only language I can speak.

For centuries, in certain rural villages of the Jiangyong region in the Hunan province of China, a secret women's language existed. It was called nüshu and was passed down through generations of women in the form of embroidered shawls, vases, and hidden writing on the inner folds of paper fans. This discreet calligraphy was the only way they could communicate at the margins of the male gaze, so often violent and imposing, which treated their writing as no more than abstract sketches, like the tracks of birds' feet in snow.

How is the mother tongue transmitted? I sketch my daughter's body across my belly in slow lines, as if printing inscriptions into clay tablets.

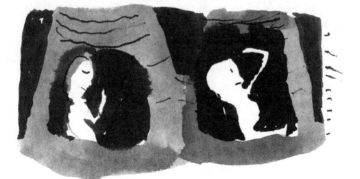

In the fourteen-week ultrasound, we see a hand, waving, with all its phalanxes extended, and an arm propped into a triangle, like someone resting on a beach chair. My daughter hasn't been born, but she's alive. Now that I've overcome the exhaustion of the first trimester, I do everything I used to do before I got pregnant, but now there are two of us. I'm living in an episode of *The Twilight Zone*: an otherworldly being takes violent possession of me, makes me disappear. As if my womb were a game of Tetris, the cells multiply and rearrange my organs.

In order to grow, my daughter consumes my allotment of breath. In this sense, she resembles the tumor that lodged in my mother's pancreas for several months. I explore the idea in all its perversion: my baby inhabits the outer reaches of what begins, and the adenocarcinoma, with its star-shaped cells (cancer is a spangled sky), inhabits the outer reaches of what ends. We welcome the former with bibs and onesies; we try to annihilate the latter with chemotherapy. In both cases, though, the void takes on new forms.

When asked, "What do you wish for your son?" the cartoonist Roberto Alfredo Fontanarrosa replied, "For his friends to cheer up when they see him coming."

The photos of the Amazon, which has been ablaze for the past three weeks, blow my mind. Faced with a catastrophe of this magnitude, the desire to reproduce is an act of utter selfishness. As my mind travels these vast expanses of fire-ravaged land, I wonder if the reasons why I decided to have a child are good enough.

> *It wasn't for love of having*
>
> *children that I had a child.*
> *Rather, I simply didn't know how a person*
>
> *could cross, fully shoeless, a bed of coals*
> *and not burn, and I needed*
>
> *someone to pass this to.*

This is how Natalie Shapero answers the question *why have children?* I'm still looking for the answer.

The doctor says that my uterus is a perfect hydraulic system. To prove it, she places the head of the ultrasound device against my belly and shakes it gently. "See? The baby doesn't even notice. Your body is better than a Michelin tire."

We name her—the tiny inhabitant of the mechanical system I am—Aurelia.

I'm going to tell you what I saw at the Monterey Bay Aquarium: an enormous tank filled with *Aurelia aurita* jellyfish, floating like shoals of cotton, of parasols, of nothing. A spectacle of flowers reconfiguring themselves. Underwater mushrooms. Beating hearts. Diminutive universes in constant expansion. Water is water but it isn't water; it's a longing to change form.

Did you dream that your heart pumped blood from one end of the city to the other? Has your room turned to liquid? Does the sun have a translucent shell?

If you say it, you break, but if you don't say it, you break.

I'm the aquarium now. You're the jellyfish.

In Vitro

We don't name you because you exist; we name you so that you'll exist.

No ancient civilization could resist the allure of using imaginary lines to connect the little shining dots that appeared in the night sky. That's how I feel when I see photographs of ultrasounds, and I go too far in my explorations of that black-and-white rectangle where someone greets me with a tiny wave. Some nights, I feel a blue fire in my head, a two-dimensional cosmos that becomes real when no one looks at it. I'm the flame floating in that darkness, and even the fish recognize me as one of their own.

In Vitro

Journal from Panama: I ran over a pelican. I tasted the best watermelon of my life. I walked under the Casco Viejo sun with a maracuyá shaved ice melting in my hand. In Panama, I woke for the first time with something like a pregnant woman's belly, a rigid protuberance just below my navel that made me realize two of us could fit inside me.

We ran it over. We tasted it. We walked. We woke.

Some years from now, when my eldest nephew dies, there will be no one left who remembers my parents alive. At most, my youngest niece and my daughter will be able to recognize their faces in the photos that my brother and I will insist on showing them.

For now, I know my daughter only in images. I conjugate her in the future as I conjugate my parents in the past.

There are nights when the baby moves so violently inside me that she turns any dream into a nightmare. I'm a bottle of thick-bubbled seltzer. A tree convulsing in the wind. A machine spewing popcorn into the air. Frenzied, she reaches out her arms and legs until my womb becomes elastic, multicolored, heeding the whims of this intruder who consumes my calcium. The skin stretches so far that I can sense every part of her brief body by touch: the exact shape of her nose, her perfect ribs, the angle of her bent knees.

I struggle to imagine my embryos in the cold. In my mind, they're made of magma, simmering in their excess of possibility. Emptied of everything else, they have room only for heat. The truth is, though, they're frozen, and we're approaching the day when we'll need to decide what to do with them. I know they're not alive, but there's no way I'd willingly spend a night in the lab that stores them.

Sheila Heti says there are many ways to be a mother besides giving birth to a biological baby. *And there are children everywhere, and parents needing help everywhere, and so much work to be done.* I could, for example, adopt a child. Volunteer at an orphanage. Offer to babysit my nieces and nephews, to water my neighbor's plants when she's out of town. I can't forget that I was, during their time in chemotherapy, a mother to my own parents. *The whole world needs to be mothered. . . . That mother could be you.*

Heti also talks about the highly specific anguish experienced, as the biological clock keeps ticking, by women who aren't sure if they want to be mothers. In some cases, all it takes is to reach a certain age. Once having kids is no longer an option, you can just stop thinking about it. That's when you hear about an acquaintance—who isn't getting any younger—who was able to get pregnant with the aid of new technologies and has just given birth to a perfectly healthy baby. So the pendulum of the decision keeps swinging, ruthlessly, overhead.

Maybe the dark line that has begun to appear on my belly, that field guide à la Hansel and Gretel to help the baby reach the nipples, is a mark that signals a secret pact among women. More specifically, among my friends, who have grown so much more significant in these past months that they even look taller to me, luminous, magnified. They accompany me in my darkest hours and gift me a crib. They spend a Sunday afternoon helping me assemble it. They organize a cheese banquet to help me reach my recommended weight. They look for recipes to counteract the nausea. Unhesitatingly, they offer me an enormous box full of clothing their daughters have outgrown. They build, with their own hands, a mobile of three whales orbiting a jellyfish in the middle. Jellyfish over jellyfish.

Sometimes, walking from my apartment to the park, I tell the dog about my plans for the week or ask for her opinion on something. *What do you think?* Because she thinks: she knows me, she listens to me, and even if she doesn't understand words, she can sense my mood and respond to it. Lately I talk with the baby, too, who has become more real as a presence ever since I started to feel her moving. So that she and the dog can begin to recognize each other, I explain to them that in a few months we'll have to reinvent our lives. God knows what the neighbors think of me: a pajama-clad woman out walking with her dog before dawn, maintaining a three-voice monologue.

On those walks, I also start thinking about the birth. The first six months have been so tranquil that the ghost of future pain has grown more concrete, as if the verdict *in pain you shall bring forth children* were lurking around the corner.

Giving birth is absolutely not comparable to publishing a book, but writing one does bear some resemblance to being pregnant. Throughout the most intense months of work, you think about something obsessively. Your mind swarms with unanswered questions and your emotions run away from you. The paragraph that verged on genius at night has become absurd by morning. But you persist: you know something is taking shape. You buy the vitamins. You show up eager to revise. You write, even if the process transpires beyond you, even if most of the time you have no idea what you're doing.

In Vitro

What I choose not to say is written, too. Something is left on the edges of the photograph. I delete: I lock a glass box inside another inside another. I place a coverslip over the world and sit still inside this private cosmos. What I allow to be heard is my silence.

Simone Weil says that pain leads to growth and light, while affliction is the victim's lot. The ravages of childbirth, then, are painful, but there is no affliction in them.

What exactly is going to break in me? How will I be born with my daughter? I want to be there for all of it.

I've felt as if I were about to give birth only twice before: the day my mother died, and then, years later, my father. Being an orphan and having a child are similar in the certainty that you will be vulnerable forever. Just as orphanhood extends beyond grief, which is eventually soothed, my condition as a mother is something that has no end.

Every day I have left, I'll be a mother.
Every day I have left, I'll be an orphan.

When asked if she still hoped to become a mother after two miscarriages, a woman replied, "I already am. I am the mother of two children who are dead."

I occasionally think of the doctor who never laughed at my jokes. I'm consumed by thoughts of what prompted him to rate one embryo as the best of the lot, to choose one spermatozoon over another. Is he taking good care of my cell clusters? The embryologist is our little human god.

I heard about a woman with endometriosis who underwent seven rounds of in vitro fertilization. The first time, there was an egg that couldn't be fertilized. The second, five eggs were extracted and three embryos attained; two poor-quality embryos survived and none took. The third time, the procedure led to a biochemical pregnancy resulting in an early miscarriage. (The first pregnancy test was positive, but with insufficient human chorionic gonadotropin levels, and by the second test, the embryo had fled, like in my dream.) The fourth attempt achieved seven embryos, but two died inside her body and the other five outside, in the lab, due to a freezing error, and so on with the fifth time, the sixth, the seventh.

Watching my shape grow rounder every week, viewing our experience as something worthwhile, I know this thought is contaminated by success.

When her son was born, Sarah Manguso stopped keeping the journal she'd maintained since adolescence. *He needed me more than I needed to write about him.* That's why I write these lines before the tsunami hits.

What happens outside sleep touches sleep. The other night it was so hot that the coconut oil I keep in a jar on my nightstand had melted into a liquid by morning. The dog wouldn't stop barking, the sheets soaked through, and I dreamed of tides and ships.

The fish, all children of mine, burned on the surface of a spring that was actually a glass receptacle in a medical lab. When I woke, my palms were hot.

For a long time, I thought my penchant for minor genres, for fragments, for the small, for what happens in vitro was a defect that diverted me from major themes. A character flaw. Until I realized that my desire inhabited these miniature spaces. My life was reconfigured by an embryo that knew how to multiply, without overflowing, until it formed the organs of my daughter.

I recently read the testimony of a woman who spent years searching for her missing daughter and was finally able to hold her remains, which had been found in a clandestine mass grave. Asked what it felt like to have those bones in her arms, the mother said it was like holding a newborn baby.

In the third-trimester structural ultrasound, my child appears upside down, suspended like a bat, her head lodged into my pelvis. At the same appointment, I'm diagnosed with oligohydramnios: a condition in which there isn't enough amniotic fluid for the baby to move around and develop as she should. I begin to drink over a gallon of water a day. With my bladder reduced to the size of a tortilla, I can't walk so much as a couple of blocks before I need to pee. My body's tenant doesn't disturb me; she transforms me.

In Vitro

A question posed by Muriel Rukeyser: *What would happen if one woman told the truth about her life?*

An answer: *The world would split open.*

As I make my way toward the final pages of this book, I think of all the titles it's had, and of the possibility of keeping its true name a secret—like the Manegrians of Siberia, who would make up a name when asked to identify themselves. When someone wanted to find a member of the community, they'd refer to them by responding, "The one you're asking about is so-and-so's son."

The ancient Egyptians had two names: one large and true, a public name, and another small, playful, intimate one they'd protect to the very end.

For years, my mother's ashes were divided up among my siblings and me. Each of us had our own portion at home: a jigsaw puzzle of tiny pieces. Years later, when my father died and we decided to combine all the ashes in a single crypt, I was startled that my mother's remains were so heavy, that something so remote in time could still exert such strength. A few days after I give birth, I think about the color of those ashes, the shards of white bone mixed with gray dust: six and a half pounds of flesh, of remnants, of possibility.

Surfer

On the day of the birth—the evening of the birth, the middle of the night of the birth, the morning of the birth, that other dimension that is the birth—I unfold beyond my body and watch myself from outside, like in those astral journeys people say can happen in dreams. The boundaries between protagonist and narrator are blurred: I'm both a woman giving birth and a woman accompanying a woman giving birth.

It's all white noise at first, so much so that we manage to eat lentils for dinner and laugh, entertained, when a contraction approaches, as if it were a harmless thing. But the labor pains soon take revenge, intensifying until they turn to wily knives that seek my flesh, strain to slash it. Knives that someone has set to heat in the open fire until the metal glows red. Knives designed specifically to make a channel of me. I drag myself out into the night, disoriented. On the way to the hospital, the pain grows so ferocious that my language has lost its coordinates by the time we reach the hospital.

I can't even answer the doctor on call when she enters the room to touch me in a way that will determine how dilated I am, but my silence doesn't keep her from opening her hand inside me, drawing a stiff five-centimeter star with her fingers.

Childbirth is like the ocean, the doula says. Don't you dare turn your back to it.

The nurses ask me to mount the contractions like waves, to surf the panic. But when I feel them coming, I can't let my body go, can't breathe, can't listen to music or inhale the essential oils we've brought in my hospital bag. I freeze, petrify, and my hips open more violently.

Dying feels like a good idea, but I resist: with every spasm, my hands grip a pair of invisible oars and I row toward the future. Outside, barbs of light begin to dawn.

Then, out of nowhere, a vision, a truce: my mother and me in a snowy city. It's 2005. The cancer had invaded her pancreas by then. We stop to buy a coat at a thrift store where all the clerks are pregnant women with their bellies bared, balloons of flesh shot through with torrential veins. The only coat we find is blue. It's too big for her—there came a time when everything was too big for her—and it covers her from neck to ankle.

Abruptly, we're outside and in the distance, trudging clumsily through the snow. My mother looks like a dying celestial gleam against the landscape's white background. The opposite of a star in the clear night sky.

At some point, the image cuts out and the pain dazzles me in an uncontrollable desire to push. And that's what I do, with all my strength, daylight now fully installed outside. But many hours pass until I hear a muffled cry in the middle of our brand-new blood. Seconds after the wail, the cord still pulsing, a pair of gloves takes my daughter and places her on my chest. She weighs as much as a small melon and her skin is as translucent as a freshly caught fish. She trawls herself toward the milk with a determination that shocks me, her eyes intensely open, as if she knows something the rest of us are oblivious to. By the time they cut the umbilical cord and the pain starts to ease, I'm so broken that I can barely recognize her.

Double Aquarius

Things I was told about childbirth that turned out to be false:

The suffering is in your head.
Your baby knows how to be born.
You know how to give birth.
You can avoid the pain if you learn to control your breathing.
Holding her in your arms for the first time will be the happiest moment of your life.

There's nothing abstract about giving birth. Everything happens in the realm of the all-too-real: the contractions that sunder you, the vaginal touch that determines the dilation of your cervix, the rotation and engagement, the head covered in black hair that peeks out of you, the gardener's shears for the episiotomy, the needle that puts the two halves of you back together, the stubborn vomiting. And throughout the entire process, a pain so colossal that it needs a new name. Yet many women remember birth as a blurry, almost faded experience.

Then the sinking, the days of colostrum, of recognizing the predawn colors, of learning to do everything one-handed. Days of sharpening the machetes, of following the river blindfolded.

What relief I would feel to visit my children's grave! says the protagonist of a novel by Luisa Josefina Hernández I read in pieces while the baby sleeps. *What peace to know I haven't had them!* For a moment, between diapers and spilled milk, I set the book aside to savor this envy.

Something ends and something begins in that hospital room, but I'm not sure what. The easiest thing would be to start from the beginning, but the beginning means nothing without what came later, and what came later means nothing without the end. I wish I didn't have to put this story's events in order. I'd rather tell all the parts at the same time, one on top of the other and another and another until the words jumble together and turn into blocks of ink, nothing more.

Maybe the last line of this book is the first of another, the start of something that doesn't belong to me and which I therefore don't attempt to define.

How can you narrate a spiral?

On February 1, 2020, as I was giving birth in Mexico City, forty-six people in China died of COVID-19. That same day, Spain reported its first national case: a German tourist isolated in a hospital on the Canary Islands. The news was still reaching us in a hazy light: twenty-seven more days would pass before the first case was confirmed in Mexico, and over six weeks before the first death. In the hospital room where my daughter and I found ourselves face-to-face for the first time, it was impossible to imagine what was coming.

What I feel is called grief. It's called sleeplessness. The scream of the mandrake. Seeing myself in a tiny body's blood. Minuscule fingernails of my flesh on other hands. The unexpected weight of an anticipated presence. Energy dragging itself like an animal behind the walls.

A silent war. My body is the battlefield.

I wanted to yank the thorns from my perineum, hide beneath a translucent veil, stick my head in an oven. Just briefly, not too long. Just enough to silence the noise and think about the possibilities for rebuilding a realm of firm muscles and plans for later.

It's called grief, except I don't know exactly what I'm losing.

My daughter's body has imposed its rhythm on the other inhabitants of our household. We move more cautiously, as if discovering the tranquil rhythms of baking, the slow softening of carrots and potatoes. The dog doesn't understand what kind of creature we've invited to live with us, but she protects her anyway, and even the plants brighten when the baby looks at them.

Our dreams are a second life, writes Gérard de Nerval in the first line of *Aurelia* before he proceeds to delve into invisible worlds, cavernous transparencies, and social gatherings where the faces of distant relatives are transformed. Motherhood is a similar delirium. Will these socks fit her? Is she still hungry? Is she stirring in her sleep? Overnight, I acquire the gift of omnipresence: wherever I am, I'm always with her. Aurelia is a second life.

Hokusai's wave is still pinned to our refrigerator, which is now full of food prepared to survive the end of the world. The magnet still holds up the image of the second ultrasound, the one with the tiny waving hand. I could replace it with a more recent photo, but I'm superstitious, and this story depends on that weathered paper. The jellyfish, with its passion for change, could abruptly turn into something else: from a small, possum-eyed mammal to a shoddy embryo that fails to multiply, fails to implant itself, fails to be born, fails.

As tenaciously as I used to check online forums for pregnant women, I now read the news on my phone. I have a
weakness for fake images of animals taking over landscapes
cleared of human beings: dolphins in the canals of Venice,
orangutans learning to wash their hands, drunk elephants
napping in a tea plantation. *Who cares if it's false,* says José
Luis Espejo. *What matters to me is proving people's need to
reconcile with the world when they no longer have any idea how.*

And I have no idea how.

I've invited my daughter to live in a place that's changing
in ways I can't grasp and I'm not the interpreter she needs.
My only wish is for time to pass quickly. For the night to
find us alive. For sleep to come so that I can dare to imagine a happy life. A better life. My own.

In motherhood, a woman exchanges her public significance for a range of private meanings, says Rachel Cusk. No matter how ready a woman may be, the transformation is radical and abrupt: everything that has happened to her from her own birth until giving birth takes on new meaning. A baby promises a future, it's true, but also alters the past and rewrites it altogether. This is why having children doesn't just separate us from the world; it separates us from ourselves.

It's no exaggeration to say that my daughter's presence reconfigured me. During gestation, due to the phenomenon of microchimerism, some fetal cells crossed the placental barrier and dispersed in me, creating a new being with the head of a lion and the body of a goat. Science hasn't yet determined what these microscopic child-bits do to the mother's body. According to some theories, their regenerative power is such that they can even repair certain cardiopathies. What's more, some evidence indicates that, postpartum, these cells encourage the production of milk and contribute to the scarring process. Fetal cells have also been found in tumors, so they may even play a part in the emergence of cancer.

I'm under construction, as if I were the newborn. I've become my daughter's daughter, somehow.

In Vitro

I can still smell the amniotic fluid in my dreams.

The images of the future that repeated themselves in my memory during pregnancy have lost their meaning: Aurelia at her grandparents' house on Sundays; Aurelia surrounded by balloons on her first birthday; Aurelia in her elementary school uniform, hair neatly combed, looking at the camera; teenage Aurelia, finding reasons to hate me. Now I can only think of her as the baby she is, with her knees and her elbows and her milky feet.

Days are where we live, says a Philip Larkin poem I murmur to myself like a mantra. *They are to be happy in,* it continues, with irresistible candor, before asking, resigned: *Where can we live but days?*

If Larkin had lived through this pandemic, perhaps the poem would say, *The moment is where we live.*

I've never felt so close to anyone as I feel to my daughter, and yet everything about her is a mystery to me. How can I possibly be the home country of this unfamiliar person: my bloodstream her river system, my heartbeat the bell that marks her official hours, my mood her weather forecast, the rumble of my intestines her native tongue?

Since she was born, we've stopped speaking the same language, but when she stirs and moves her arms as if conducting an invisible orchestra, that music sounds for both of us with the force of a memory from another life. After nine months of laying the bricks, it's time to learn how to name the walls that divide us. To invent a vocabulary for loving each other.

Childbirth is the shipwreck in an enormous fish tank that soon shatters and populates the world around it. What world? One with no maps, and which I travel not as a mother, but as a daughter of myself.

Acknowledgments

Thanks to the women who took care of my daughter while I wrote this book: Irma, Sofía, Tanya, Antonia, and Karen. You'll never know how much your company sustained me.

Thanks to Dr. Alexandra Bermúdez, whose voice brought me back in the early hours of February 1, 2020, and thanks to Jonathan Silva for helping me color-code the clothes of language.

Thanks to Emilio Hinojosa for the landscape transformed and shared. For the curls.

Almadía first trusted in this book, and Coffee House Press gave it a home away from home; I'm deeply grateful for that. To Robin Myers, my translator and beloved friend, my ongoing gratitude and admiration.

Coffee House Press began as a small letterpress operation in 1972 and has grown into an internationally renowned nonprofit publisher of literary fiction, essay, poetry, and other work that doesn't fit neatly into genre categories.

Coffee House is both a publisher and an arts organization. Through our *Books in Action* program and publications, we've become interdisciplinary collaborators and incubators for new work and audience experiences. Our vision for the future is one where a publisher is a catalyst and connector.

LITERATURE
is not the same thing as
PUBLISHING

Funder Acknowledgments

Coffee House Press is an internationally renowned independent book publisher and arts nonprofit based in Minneapolis, MN; through its literary publications and *Books in Action* program, Coffee House acts as a catalyst and connector—between authors and readers, ideas and resources, creativity and community, inspiration and action.

Coffee House Press books are made possible through the generous support of grants and donations from corporations, state and federal grant programs, family foundations, and the many individuals who believe in the transformational power of literature. This activity is made possible by the voters of Minnesota through a Minnesota State Arts Board Operating Support grant, thanks to the legislative appropriation from the Arts and Cultural Heritage Fund. Coffee House also receives major operating support from the Amazon Literary Partnership, Jerome Foundation, Literary Arts Emergency Fund, McKnight Foundation, and the National Endowment for the Arts (NEA). To find out more about how NEA grants impact individuals and communities, visit www.arts.gov.

Coffee House Press receives additional support from Bookmobile; Dorsey & Whitney LLP; Elmer L. & Eleanor J. Andersen Foundation; the Gaea Foundation; the Matching Grant Program Fund of the Minneapolis Foundation; Mr. Pancks' Fund in memory of Graham Kimpton; the Schwab Charitable Fund; and the U.S. Bank Foundation.

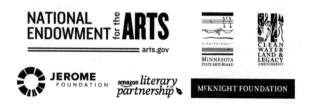

The Publisher's Circle of Coffee House Press

Publisher's Circle members make significant contributions to Coffee House Press's annual giving campaign. Understanding that a strong financial base is necessary for the press to meet the challenges and opportunities that arise each year, this group plays a crucial part in the success of Coffee House's mission.

Recent Publisher's Circle members include many anonymous donors, Patricia A. Beithon, Anitra Budd, Andrew Brantingham, Kelli & Dave Cloutier, Mary Ebert & Paul Stembler, Kamilah Foreman, Eva Galiber, Jocelyn Hale & Glenn Miller Charitable Fund of the Minneapolis Foundation, the Rehael Fund-Roger Hale/Nor Hall of the Minneapolis Foundation, Randy Hartten & Ron Lotz, Dylan Hicks & Nina Hale, William Hardacker, Kenneth & Susan Kahn, the Kenneth Koch Literary Estate, Cinda Kornblum, Jennifer Kwon Dobbs & Stefan Liess, the Lenfestey Family Foundation, Rebecca Rand, Sarah Lutman & Rob Rudolph, the Carol & Aaron Mack Charitable Fund of the Minneapolis Foundation, Gillian McCain, Mary & Malcolm McDermid, Robin Chemers Neustein, Daniel N. Smith III & Maureen Millea Smith, Enrique & Jennifer Olivarez, Robin Preble, Nan G. Swid, Grant Wood, and Margaret Wurtele.

For more information about the Publisher's Circle and other ways to support Coffee House Press books, authors, and activities, please visit www.coffeehousepress.org/pages/donate or contact us at info@coffeehousepress.org.

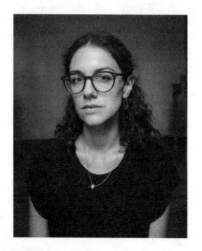

Isabel Zapata was born in Mexico City in 1984. She is the author of *Las noches son así, Alberca vacía / Empty Pool* (translated by Robin Myers), and *Una ballena es un país*. In 2015, she and four friends founded the press Ediciones Antílope.

Robin Myers is a poet and Spanish-to-English translator. Her translations include *Salt Crystals* by Cristina Bendek (Charco Press), *Copy* by Dolores Dorantes (Wave Books), *The Dream of Every Cell* by Maricela Guerrero (Cardboard House Press), *The Book of Explanations* by Tedi López Mills (Deep Vellum Publishing), and *The Restless Dead* by Cristina Rivera Garza (Vanderbilt University Press), among other works of poetry and prose. She was double-longlisted for the 2022 National Translation Award in poetry. She lives in Mexico City.

In Vitro was designed by
Bookmobile Design & Digital Publisher Services.
Text is set in Freight Text Pro.